Joe learns About Fabry Disease

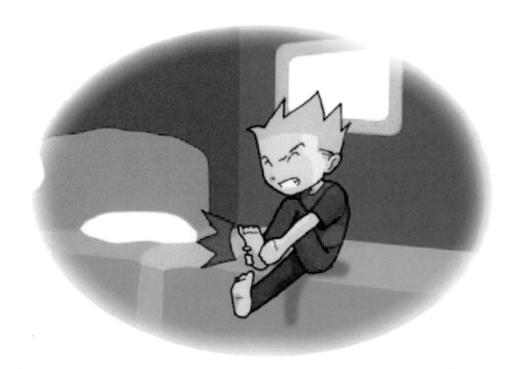

Written by Dawn Laney, MS
Illustrated by Michael Johnson

ISBN: 1-4392-4584-3
EAN13: 9781439245842
LCCN: 2009905921

Visit www.booksurge.com or contact the Emory Lysosomal Storage Disease Center
at 404-778-8565 to order additional copies.

Joe was published with the assistance of an educational grant from Genzyme Corporation.

Revenue from the sale of this book will be used to support the Emory Lysosomal Storage Disease Center.

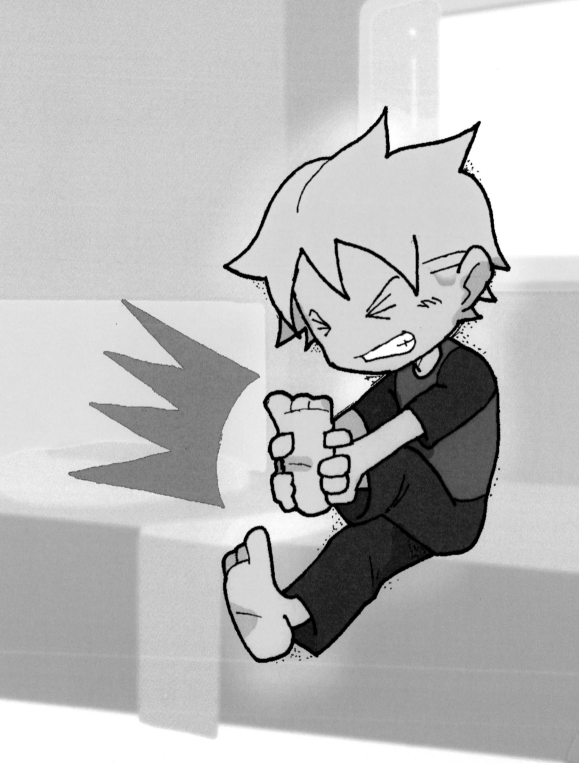

Joe woke up late one morning feeling
grumpy and down in the dumps.
Yesterday he had had a great day running
and playing with his friends outside, but this
morning his feet were hurting AGAIN.

OW! OW! OW!

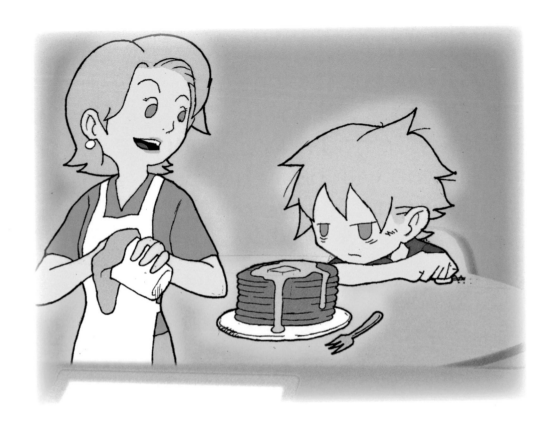

He went downstairs to breakfast. Even the
sight of a stack of pancakes dripping with
butter and syrup didn't make him smile.

"Why so grouchy Joe?" his mother said.

Joe looked at his mother and
growled "I'm not grouchy."

Joe's mother sat down and looked at him closely. "Joe, are your feet hurting again?"

At first, Joe didn't want to talk about it, but his mother looked a little worried, so he said, "Yeah, they hurt again. Why do my feet hurt? I didn't bump them or drop a rock on them or anything!"

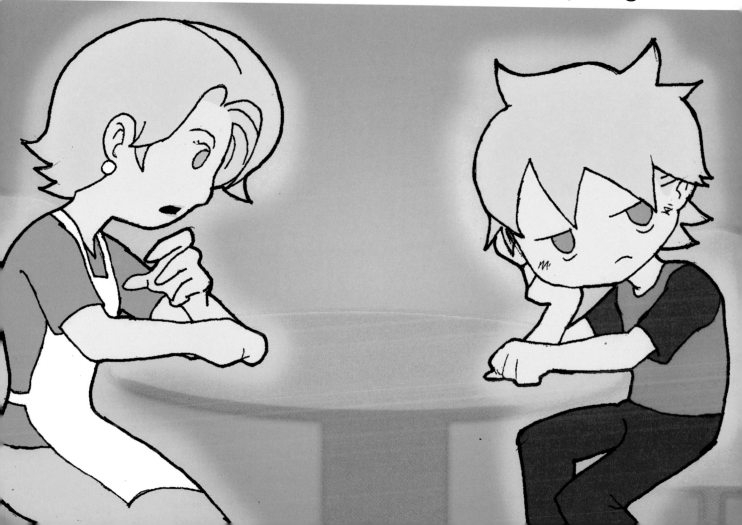

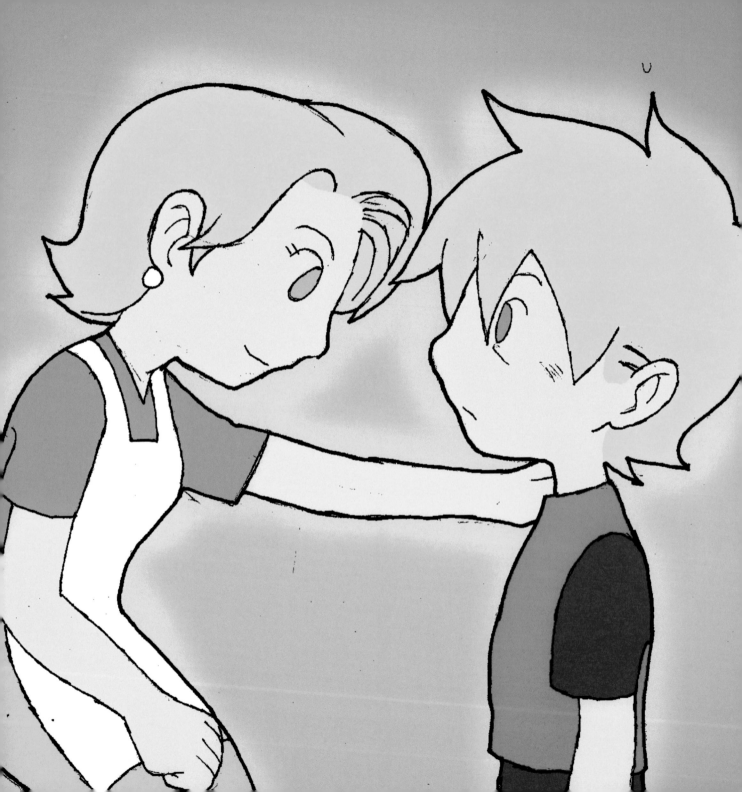

Joe's mother said, "I know you didn't do anything to make them hurt. We are going to a special doctor today to talk with him about your feet and your stomach pain too."

Joe was not excited to go to the doctor. He had been to so many doctors already.

Joe's mother reassured him that this doctor was a genetic doctor and had heard of other people like Joe with foot pain. She said that hopefully the doctor would be able to tell him why his feet hurt and then make it stop.

After breakfast, Joe and his mother went to the big red building where the doctor worked.

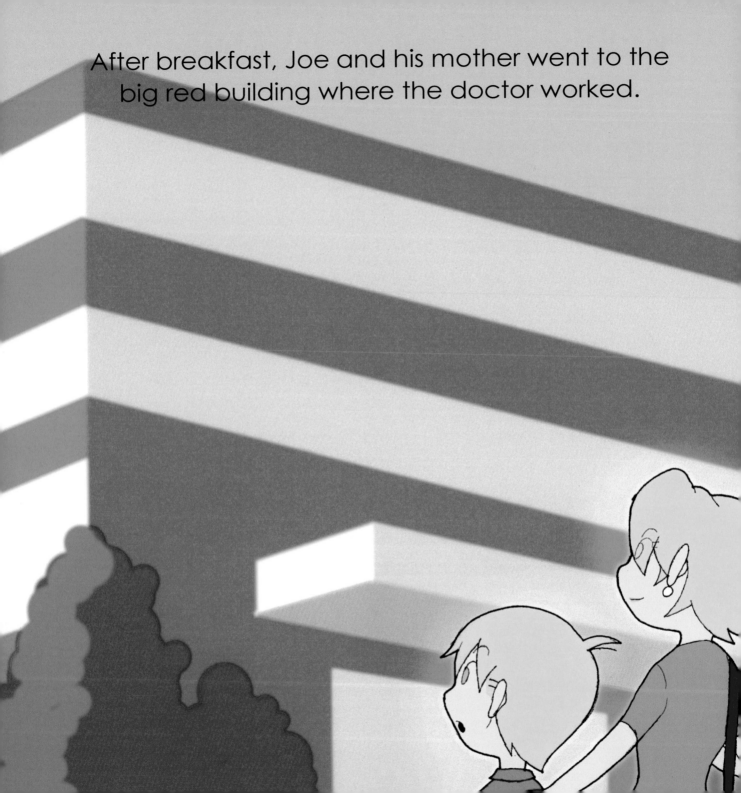

At the doctor's office, there was a window for Joe's mother to sign in and a waiting room filled with fun books and toys.

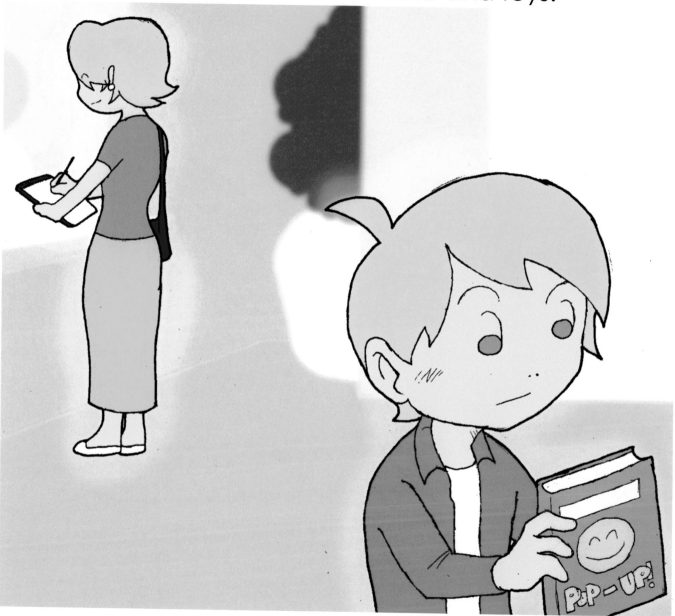

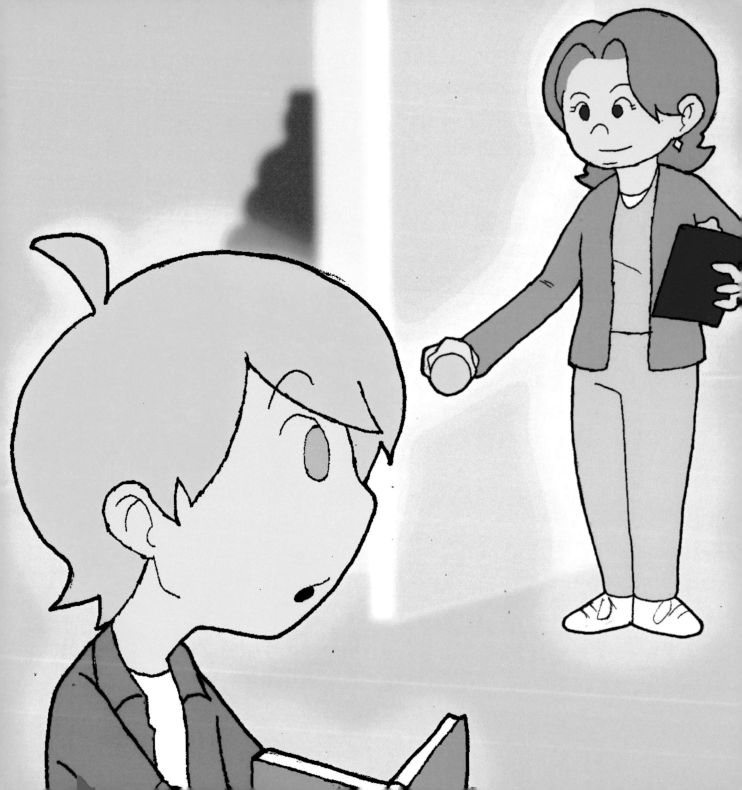

Soon a nurse in brightly colored clothes called Joe's name and asked them to follow her. "Hi!" the nurse said as they walked, "I'm Angela and I'm going to take your temperature, see how tall you are, and see how much you weigh."

Then the nurse took Joe and his mother into a little room with a paper covered table and some chairs.

Soon, a nice lady came to talk
with Joe and his mother.

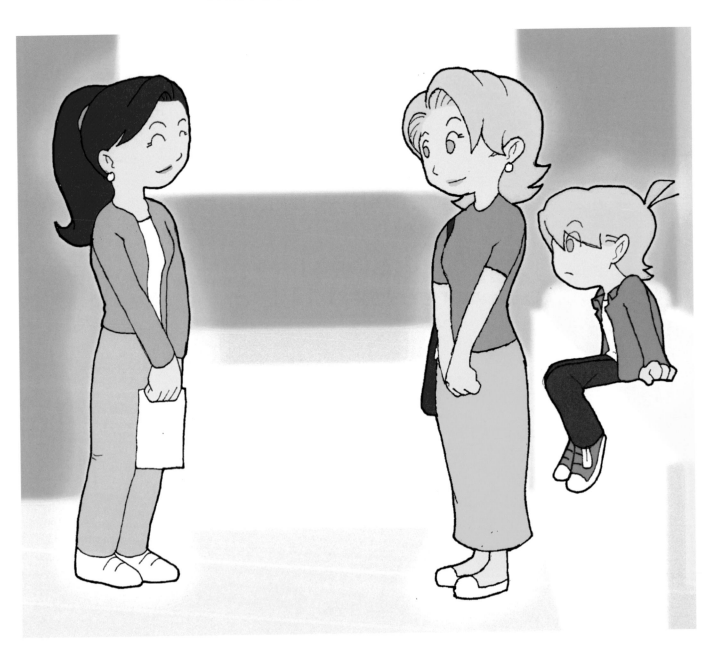

"Hello Joe," the woman said, "I'm Mary the genetic counselor. I am here to ask you and your mom some questions about those pains in your feet and other things you might be feeling."

Joe was a little shy at first, but soon he was answering all of Mary's questions before his mother could even open her mouth to reply. Some of her questions were funny and about things like sweating and gym class.

Next a cheerful doctor came into the room
"Good morning young man," the doctor said,

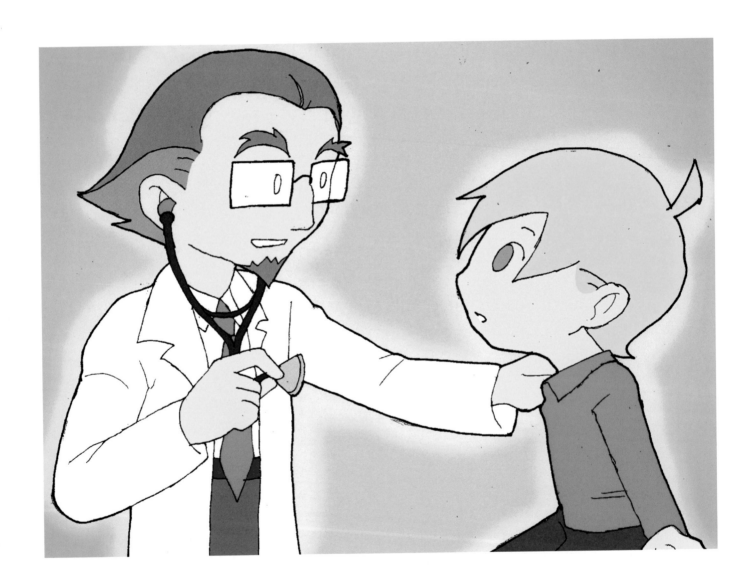

"I'm Dr. Fisher. Mary has told me all about you and I'm very glad to meet you. I think I have the answer to why your feet hurt, but I'd like to take a look at you first if that is OK with you."

Joe looked at his mother, who nodded that it was OK. Joe hopped up on the table covered with paper. After Dr. Fisher listened to Joe's heart and felt Joe's belly (which tickled!), Dr. Fisher asked Joe about school and his friends.

Joe told Dr. Fisher about the weird feeling he had a lot in his hands and feet, like they were asleep or covered in sand. He also talked about how tired he got during gym class and recess. He often had to stop playing, even though he really wanted to keep going.

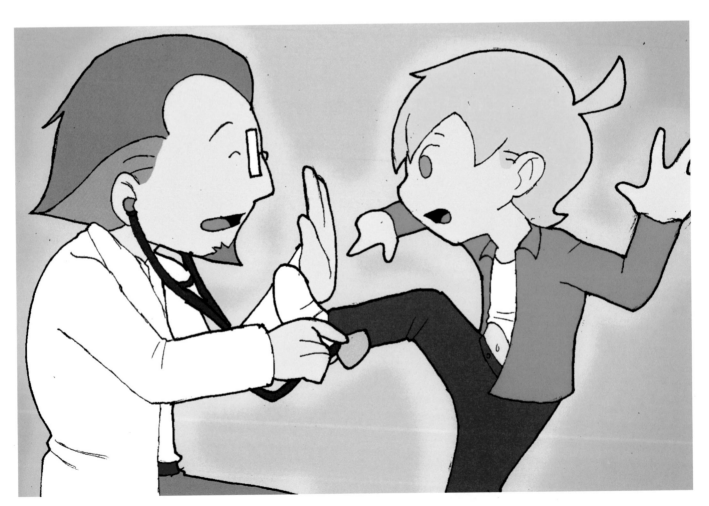

At the end of the visit, Dr. Fisher asked Joe if it would be OK if he had the nurse take a little of his blood from his arm using a needle.

Joe was afraid, but Dr. Fisher explained that it would only be a little of his blood and that Joe would have plenty left. He also said that they could use a special cream on his arm before using the needle. That way it wouldn't hurt as much.

Joe was nervous, but he was brave and said "OK."

The nurse came back in and put a cool cream on Joe's arm. She waited a little while and then collected some of Joe's blood using a needle. It was done in no time! Joe's mother was very proud of him and Joe got to pick a sticker to take home. He chose a sticker with a picture of his favorite superhero on it.

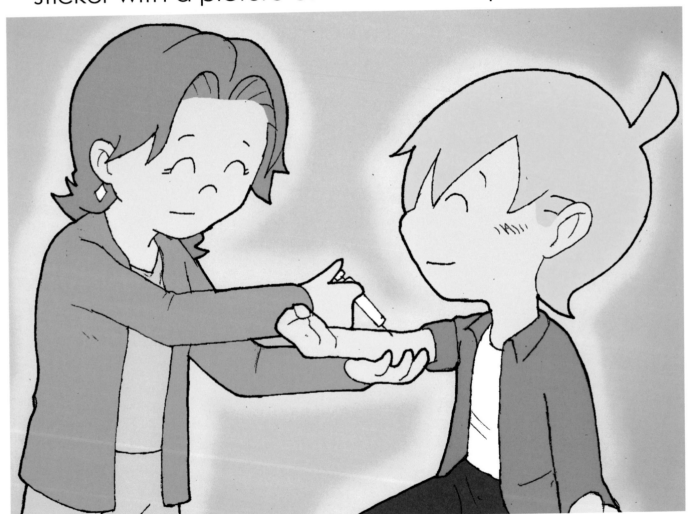

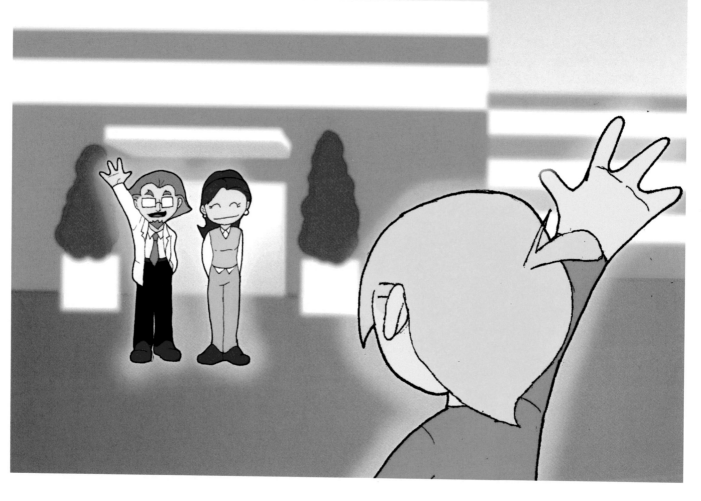

Two weeks later, Joe and his parents went back to the little red building to talk with Dr. Fisher and Mary again. Dr. Fisher and Mary talked to Joe's parents for a little while, and then they talked directly to Joe.

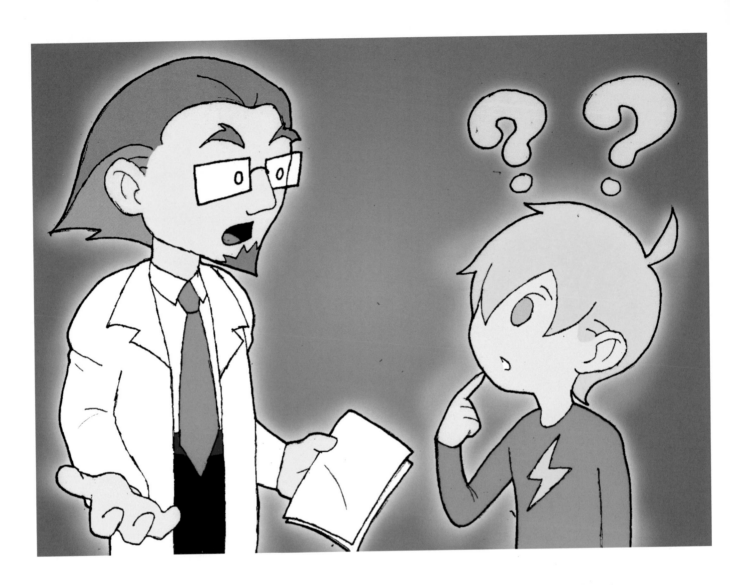

"Hey Joe," Dr. Fisher said, "Do you remember that blood you let me have at your last visit?"

Joe remembered!

"Good!" Dr. Fisher said, "When we looked at your blood we looked closely at the chemicals your body uses to work. We learned that one of them is broken, and some gunk is building up in your body."

Joe wasn't quite sure what that meant
and gave Dr. Fisher a puzzled look.

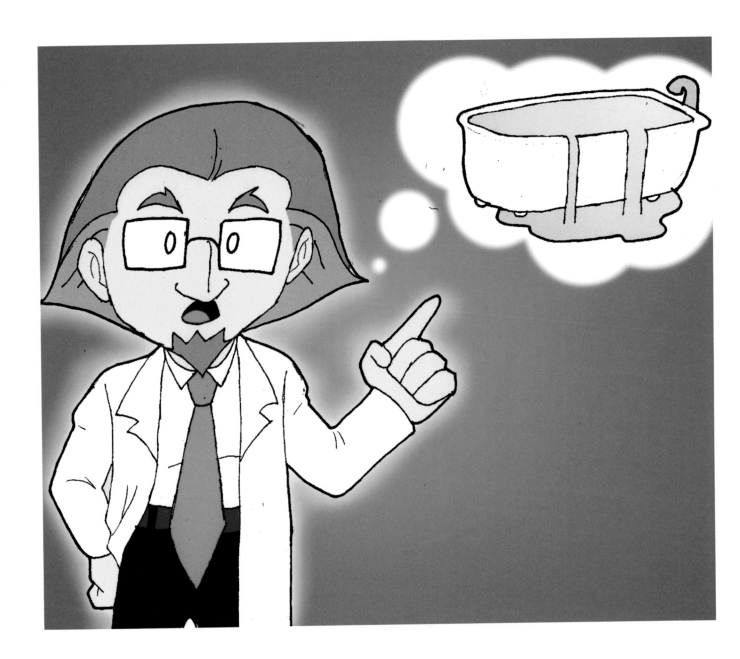

"Think of it a different way. Pretend that your body is a bath tub. In order to keep the bath tub clean and ready for your baths, you need a drain that works. If the drain is clogged, the bath tub will overflow spilling water all over the bathroom and making a mess. Just like a bathtub with a clogged drain, your body is building up gunk and it causes your feet and stomach to hurt."

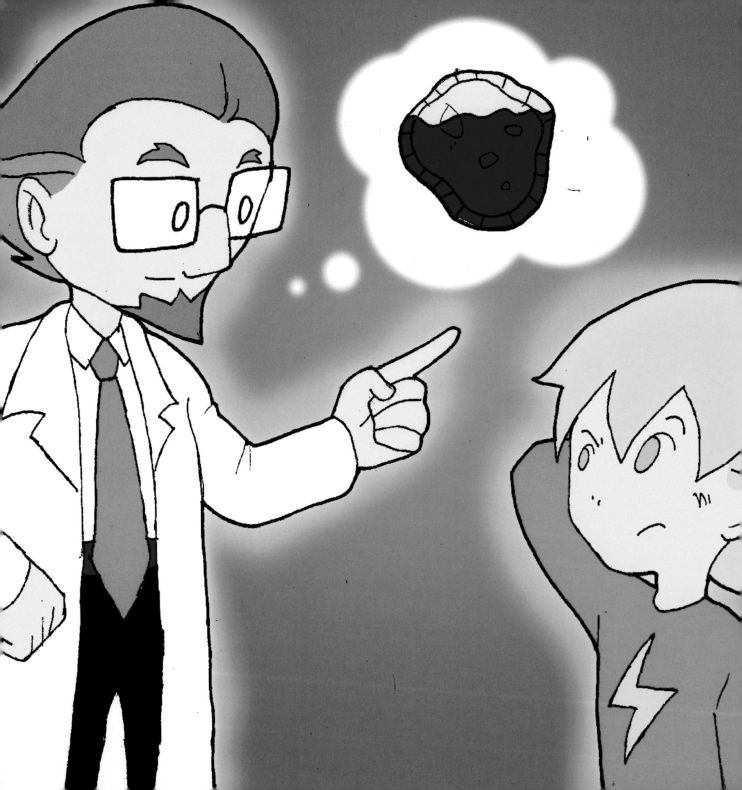

Overflowing bathtubs made sense to Joe;
he had done that a few times at his house.
But, what did that mean for him and his feet?

Dr. Fisher didn't let Joe wonder for long. "Joe,"
he said, "It is called Fabry disease when your
body has this kind of gunk building up inside it."

"fa-BRAY" Joe thought, that's a weird name.

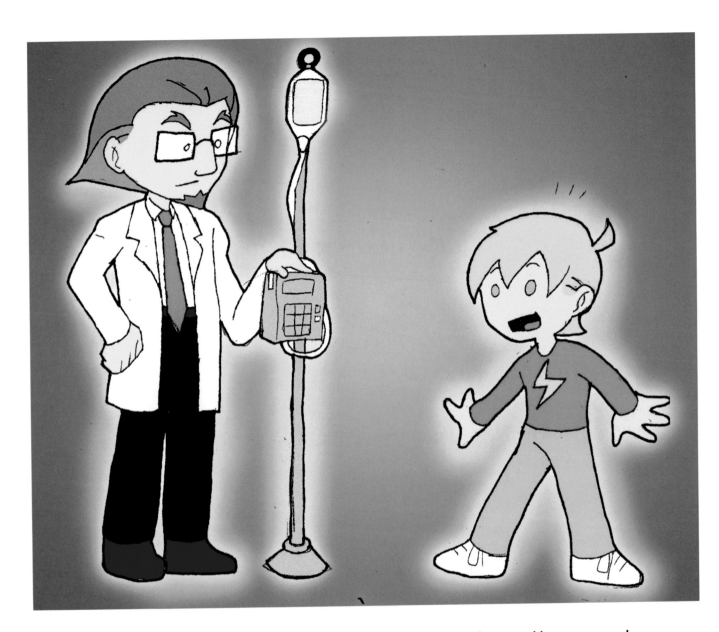

Dr. Fisher continued, "We can clear the gunk
out of your body and make you feel better
using a special kind of medicine."

Joe was relieved; he did want to feel better. "When can I start?!" he said.

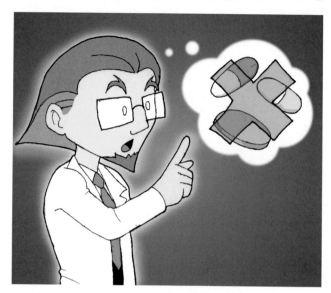

"Soon," Dr. Fisher said, "But it is important for you to know that this medicine is not like your vitamins. This medication we put directly into your blood with a needle. This is called an infusion."

Joe looked at his parents; he didn't like needles. Dr. Fisher explained that he would only need the medicine twice a month and that they could use the cream every time so that he wouldn't feel the needle.

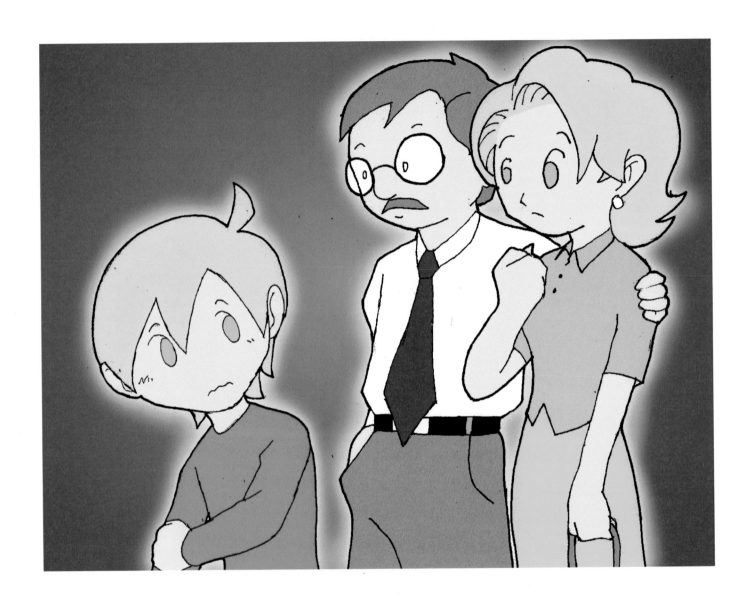

Joe thought hard about his hurting feet, his belly aches, and being so tired. He knew that if the medicine could fix those things, he wanted to do it. Joe told his parents that he would try it. HOWEVER, he definitely wanted the no-hurt cream.

His parents smiled and said they understood. Then Dr. Fisher, Mary, and his parents talked for a while about schedules and timing.

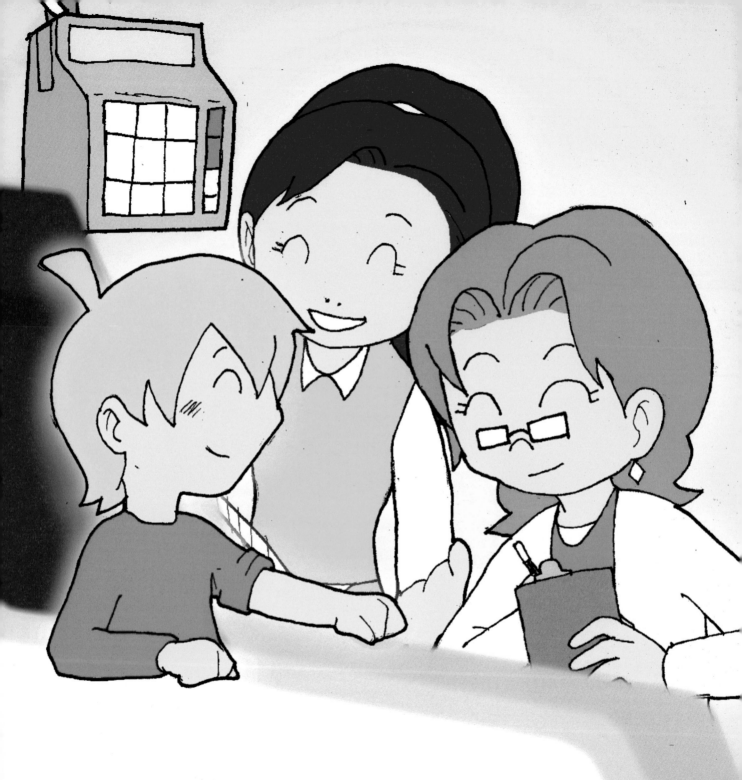

Joe did go and get his medicine. At first, he was a little scared and nervous before each visit, but Angela, the nice nurse, always explained everything that she was doing and he got to watch movies while he got his medicine.

Joe also met other kids who were getting their medicine at the same time he was. They had a good time talking and playing games together.

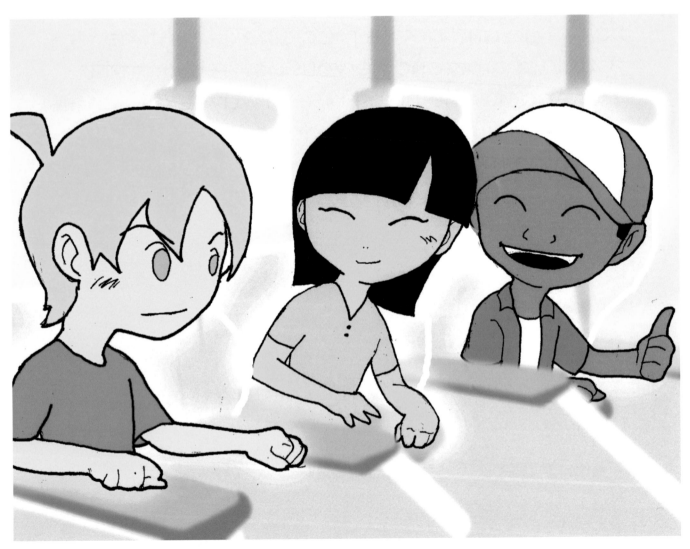

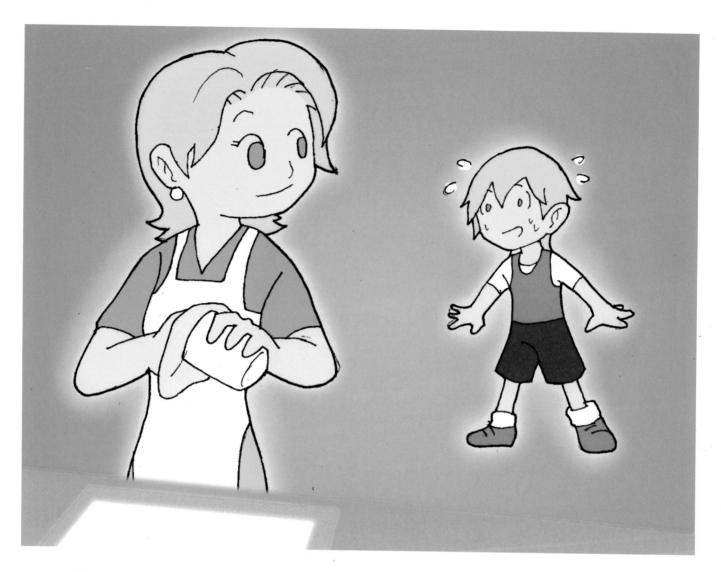

After a little while, Joe told his mother that he had started sweating when he was hot. He also could keep up with his friends at recess and in gym. In fact, Joe had won the relay race on Field day!

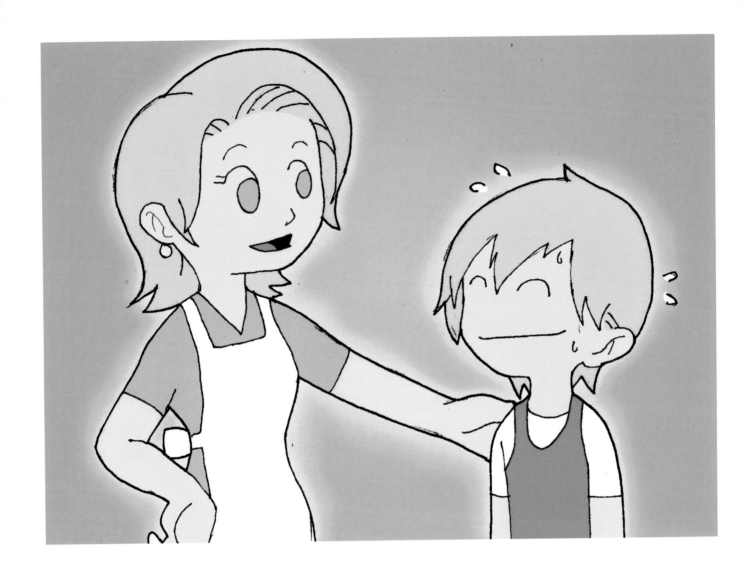

Joe's mother also reminded him that he hadn't mentioned his feet and stomach hurting in a long time.

Joe thought about it and said, "You are right, I haven't hurt in a while."
"This means no more bad, grumpy days!" Joe said.

"Well, maybe a few grumpy days," his mother said with a smile, "but not because of sore feet."

Dawn Laney is genetic counselor and research coordinator at the Emory Lysosomal Storage Disease Center. She works closely with families affected by Fabry disease and other related conditions. She spends her free time playing with her son, painting, hiking, reading, and writing children's books.

Michael Johnson is an illustrator and graphic artist living in the Atlanta, Georgia area. His loves are designing video games and staying cool. He knows Joe's pain first hand as he happens to be affected by Fabry disease.

Emory's Lysosomal Storage Disease Center in Atlanta, Georgia provides diagnostic, evaluation, management, and treatment services for patients from all over the United States.

The Center is devoted to remaining on the cutting edge of research and treatment providing comprehensive and compassionate care for all of our patients affected by lysosomal storage diseases such as Fabry disease.

To speak with a member of our lysosomal storage disease team, call 404-778-8565 or 800-200-1524 visit our website at http://genetics.emory.edu/LSDC/lsdc.php.

Note:

Joe's story was developed to help explain Fabry disease and its treatment from the perspective of a ten year old. Children affected by Fabry disease can have different symptoms and response to therapy than those that Joe describes. Common symptoms of Fabry disease in childhood can include: a purplish-pink skin rash, decreased sweating, fatigue, diarrhea, headaches, frequent overheating, protein in the urine, and burning or tingling pain in their hands and/or feet.

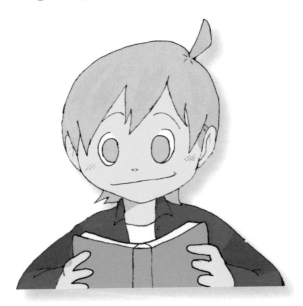

For more information about the symptoms or treatment of Fabry disease, please contact the Emory Lysosomal Storage Disease Center at 800-200-1524 or visit our website at

http://genetics.emory.edu/LSDC/lsdc.php.

Additional resources can be found at the Fabry Support and Information Group (http://www.fabry.org) and the National Fabry Disease Foundation (http://www.thenfdf.org)